How To Apply Makeup Like A Professional

Best Tips And Tricks For Makeup Application

By: Lisa Patrick

TABLE OF CONTENTS

PUBLISHERS NOTES

Disclaimer

This publication is intended to provide helpful and informative material. It is not intended to diagnose, treat, cure, or prevent any health problem or condition, nor is intended to replace the advice of a physician. No action should be taken solely on the contents of this book. Always consult your physician or qualified health-care professional on any matters regarding your health and before adopting any suggestions in this book or drawing inferences from it.

The author and publisher specifically disclaim all responsibility for any liability, loss or risk, personal or otherwise, which is incurred as a consequence, directly or indirectly, from the use or application of any contents of this book.

Any and all product names referenced within this book are the trademarks of their respective owners. None of these owners have sponsored, authorized, endorsed, or approved this book.

Always read all information provided by the manufacturers' product labels before using their products. The author and publisher are not responsible for claims made by manufacturers.

© **2013**

Manufactured in the United States of America

DEDICATION

This book is dedicated to all women who want to learn how to apply their makeup flawlessly.

CHAPTER 1- BEFORE APPLYING MAKEUP- THE TOOLS THAT ARE REQUIRED

If you often find that your makeup just doesn't look right or doesn't last as long as it should, it's possible that you may not be taking the appropriate steps before applying it. There are certain tools and techniques that you need to take advantage of before you even begin to apply your makeup. These tools and techniques have long been closely protected industry trade secrets, but the internet has made knowledge readily available for those that are interested in learning more about the best way to apply their makeup and get an airbrushed, glowing effect.

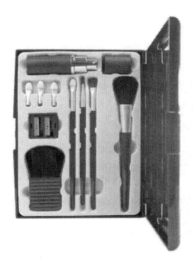

Where to Get the Tools

Most of the tools that you will need before applying your makeup will be available through your local beauty care store or through the internet at extremely affordable and reasonable prices. As always, you may wish to check the reviews of each product that you use before investing in it because all products are different. There are always cheap, grocery store brands of products as well as luxury brands, but being a luxury brand doesn't automatically make something better.

Face Wash

If you're not washing your face directly before applying your makeup, you're already doing something wrong. Oils and debris that can build up on your face will easily botch even the best makeup job. Even if you just got out of the shower in the morning, you should use a good face wash to prepare your skin for the makeup. Washing your face will help your makeup adhere to your skin and will prevent you from breaking out afterwards. A good face wash is a necessity in every woman's arsenal, and using ordinary soap to wash your face simply won't cut it.

Toner

Once you've washed your face, it's time for toner. Toner does a few things before you put on your makeup: it gets rid of any excess oil left by the face wash, it cleans up any face wash you may have missed, it refines your pores and it picks up any additional debris. Toner can also be instrumental in helping those with skin problems fight off acne and other skin issues. Most brands of skin care provide an excellent toner that can be used to treat and perfect your skin.

BB Cream

Beauty Balm has recently become a very popular way to prime your face for makeup. BB cream fills in any imperfections in your skin and can also add affects such as changing your skin color or adding a reflective, glimmering appearance. There are many BB creams available, and you can select the cream that works well for you. Many BB creams are also slightly tinted, which helps with foundation coverage.

Kabuki Brush

A kabuki brush is a necessary tool in any woman's makeup box. A kabuki brush is the best way to apply face powder, mineral powder, blush or bronzer. Using a kabuki brush creates that perfect airbrushed finish that most people are looking for, without any harsh lines or missed spots.

Eye Primer

Eye shadow primer is a simple cream that goes over your eyelids. It does two things: it makes eye shadow last longer without creasing, and it provides a deeper and bolder color. Eye shadow primer is available through many makeup lines, and some of it is even colored to add a bolder or cleaner look.

Lip Liner

If you aren't sure why your lipstick isn't looking the way it does in the magazines, it's very likely that you decided to skip the step of lip liner. Many girls today avoid lip liner because it feels unnecessary or because they think that it doesn't matter, but it truly does. Lip liner allows you to change the appearance of your lips, avoid smudging and avoid bleeding. The best lip liner to use will be the same brand as your lipstick, as it will have been specially formulated to work well with it.

Eye Shadow Brush Set

If you notice that you have quite a lot of problems applying your eye shadow, it might not be your fault. You might simply not be using the right brushes. There are very specific brushes that need to be used to apply make up in the right fashion. A larger brush is used for the brow, a mid-sized brush is used for the eye lids and an angled brush is usually used for accents and creases. A comprehensive eye shadow brush set is very likely to make your life a lot easier.

Setting Spray

Many brands of cosmetics offer a finishing spray. Finishing sprays are a simple liquid spray that will set your makeup and give it a smooth and matte appearance. If you want your makeup to last, you should always use a finishing spray. One important thing to note is that a finishing spray should seldom be sprayed directly on your face. Instead, you will usually want to mist the area in front of your face and then gently wave the spray towards your skin. Otherwise, the experience might be a little too intense.

Makeup

Of course, it goes without saying that you will also want to have a comprehensive set of makeup: eye shadow, blush, foundation, eye liner, lipstick, lip gloss, mascara, brow definers and bronzer are all essential for those seeking that fashion magazine look. While it may seem a little overwhelming at first, applying makeup the correct way will become easier and faster each time.

CHAPTER 2- MAKEUP APPLICATION- THE IMPORTANCE OF KNOWING SKIN TYPE

Whether you have been wearing makeup for years or you are just getting acquainted with various products, you probably have a sense that there are some "rules" you should follow. While makeup is definitely a creative domain, you absolute need to know about your skin type before you purchase products. Here are some of the reasons why.

Oily Skin

This is the perfect place to start because it presents an issue that so many people deal with on a regular basis. When you have oily skin, you are probably prone to breakouts. By putting certain types of makeup on your face, you are increasing the chances for even more issues with acne. Some say you cannot wear makeup at all because the products will not allow your skin to breathe. Fortunately, this is not true. Many brands make products that are specifically designed for individuals who have oily skin.

Dry Skin

On the other end of the spectrum, we have individuals who tend to experience an array of issues with dry skin. Just as makeup can make oily skin oilier, makeup can also make dry skin drier. First, you need to choose products that are designed for people who have dry skin. However, you also need to be sure you are moisturizing. You can still get acne with dry skin, so do not go overboard with the moisturizing products. Instead, choose one that is designed for the face and apply it once or twice per day. With dry skin, twice is usually better.

Combination Skin

Ah, so you are one of the lucky ones! Or so you think. When you have combination skin, you might not think it matters which type of makeup you use since your skin is a perfect blend of both. Although it might be a blend, you can still experience some problems. For example, let's say that you purchase products that are intended for people with oily skin. Since you are now going too far in one direction, you may actually end up with drier skin. Look for products that are specifically designed for individuals with combination skin.

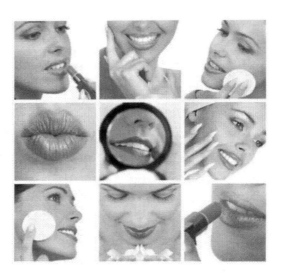

Skin Type: The Color Subset

When we are discussing skin type, terms such as "oily," "dry" and "combination" is very important. However, please remember that color is part of your skin type as well. Choosing the wrong color for certain makeup items, especially for foundation and loose powder, can be disastrous. If you opt for a shade that is too light, you may not have any coverage for the imperfections on your skin at all. Shades that are too dark are equally as problematic as they can make your skin appear orange or dirty.

Problems with Red Areas

So many people have red areas on their skin, and they do not know how to tackle them. Of course, you should also discuss these issues with your doctor to ensure that it is not a serious condition. When you have some redness on your skin, you can actually use makeup to soothe it out; you just need to know which products to buy. Look for concealers and foundations that have green undertones. You might even buy a product that is green. When you use these products on your face, they help to cancel out the redness. Don't worry; the green is easily hidden with your foundation.

Allergic Reactions

As you are considering your skin type, you also need to consider what ingredients you are allergic to. Sometimes, allergic reactions do not manifest themselves right away. You might put on an eye shadow or a foundation and not realize you are allergic to it until hours later. Some people do not have troubles with allergies. If you do, you definitely need to look into the ingredients list before you put anything on your face. Just consider how close these allergens would be to your sensitive eyes, mouth, ears, nose and other body parts.

Sweating Makeup Away

Of course, knowing how much you sweat is a part of selecting and applying the right types of makeup as well. Some people do tend to sweat a lot on their faces, especially around their foreheads and right under their noises. This can have disastrous consequences for your makeup, and your face might resemble a puddle by the end of the day. If you are a person who sweats a lot, then you should look into some primers. The primers will help your makeup to stay fresh and beautiful all day long.

Working with a Professional

Perhaps you have a makeup appointment scheduled with a professional. Whether you are getting your makeup done for a wedding or just for a night out on the town, being pampered is a lot of fun. However, if you are just meeting the makeup artist for the first time, he or she does not know what your skin is like. If you come to the session under-prepared, then the results might not be what you expected. While some makeup artists may be able to tell what type of skin you have, you should be prepared to let them know as well.

As you can see, knowing your skin type is not something to take lightly when it comes to makeup. If you do not what your skin is like, then you are not going to be able to select products to give that perfect finish in photos.

CHAPTER 3- AN INTRODUCTION TO CORRECTIVE MAKEUP

When considering the use of corrective makeup, there are two common goals that people attempt to achieve. They aim to create a more proportioned facial appearance, and to conceal specific flaws or blemishes caused by a number of unavoidable circumstances. These goals can be accomplished in a number of ways. Using concealing agents, basic foundation or other shading and shadowing techniques to emphasize the face's best features is often suggested.

Obviously, depending on the specific needs of an individual, the approach will be dramatically different than someone else. For instance, someone with an angular face will likely use shading to soften features, while a rounded face might consider accenting a jaw line or enhancing cheekbones. However, by following a few guiding principles and making intelligent choices, anyone can gain the benefits of effectively using corrective makeup.

Facial Shape

The first thing to consider is the overall facial shape. In a large number of cases, the person choosing to use corrective makeup simply wants to increase the overall proportion of their face. Since the ideal shape of a face is an oval, most theories of corrective makeup involve bringing specific facial shapes more in line with this oval ideal. Here are a number of common facial shapes and a basic approach to work with each one.

Rounded Shape: If a person has full, rounded cheeks, the lower half of the face must be brought to more of a peak than it appears naturally. One way to accomplish this is through the use of darker shades of foundation. People with this issue should choose a foundation that is one to two shades darker than their typical foundation. This new, darker foundation should be applied to the lower half of the face only, and the outer edges of that region specifically. This will give the appearance of a taper, and allow the face to appear more naturally oval than before. It can also help to apply highlights to the chin, to further accentuate this peak.

Block Shape: For those with broad foreheads or strong jaw lines, accents should be placed on the center of the face. This can be accomplished through accents on the cheekbones. Central features are typically softer than the outer region of the face, so their emphasis helps soften the appearance of the entire face. Also, shading should be used liberally on the outer region of the face, with special attention given to the forehead and jaw.

Rectangular Shape: This shape is treated similar to the block shape, with special emphasis given to shade the forehead area. Since it is difficult to diminish the appearance of length on the lower half of the face, the forehead represents the best opportunity. Shading the top of the forehead, as well as choosing a hairstyle that helps diminish the prominence of the top half of the face is vital. Again, highlighting the cheekbones is a good idea for adding width to the facial appearance and to draw natural attention away from the forehead.

Heart or Triangle Shape: Dealing with this facial shape is a two-pronged approach. First, width needs to be created utilizing similar techniques to those used in the rectangular shape scenario. Highlighting cheekbones and using lighter foundation on the outer edges of the face in this area is suggested. Blush is also typically used to further accentuate the middle of the face and to diminish the aesthetic impact of the triangular face's taper. Shading of the forehead can be used, but be careful not to create a rectangular appearance.

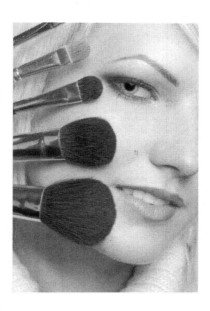

Concealing Techniques

Most people consider concealing techniques as an option for concealing blemishes. While this is true, there are a number of methods used for concealing flaws with specific facial parts as well. Since symmetry is the goal, any asymmetrical feature can be assisted with concealing techniques.

Eyes: To conceal the impact of overly round eyes, eye shadow should be extended slightly past the outer corner of the eye. This creates a point, which diminishes a round appearance. This is also a good technique for people with naturally small eyes, as it can give the illusion of size and proportion. Darker eye shadow can be used to soften overly prominent eyes, and conversely, light shadow can be used to help overcome deeper sets.

Brows: For people with rounder faces, high arched brows help give the illusion of length. However, for rectangular or triangle face shapes, this should be avoided consistently. Brows can also be trimmed short on the inner edge to create more space for people with closely set eyes. Similarly, slightly trimming the outer edge can help widely set eyes

15

appear more naturally aligned. For low foreheads, keeping the brow arch low creates a proportioned height with the forehead.

Lips: One of the most focused upon areas of the face, there are a number of tips that can help this important area stand out. For thin lips, using a lip lining pencil to outline the upper and lower lip can help create volume. However, use this sparingly, since too much pencil use can look awkward. Light lipstick also helps in this situation. For the other problem, using the lip liner just inside the lip line can actually create a less full, more proportioned appearance. Soft colors in the corners help drooping lips as well.

CHAPTER 4- HOW TO DEAL WITH IMPERFECTIONS AND BLEMISHES WHEN APPLYING MAKEUP

Having perfect skin is a blessing and for many of us we simply do not have this luxury. For those of us that have to work harder to obtain balanced and clear skin the first thing to remember is you're not alone. In this chapter, I will give you a few tips and pointers on how to deal with these imperfections and blemishes and how to deal with them when applying makeup.

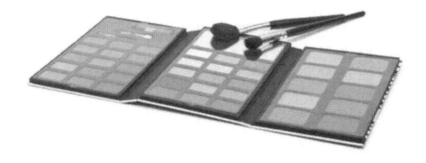

As mentioned in previous chapters the first thing you want to do before putting on your makeup is to have a clean surface to work with. I have had several problems with my skin; and I found that you don't have to spend too much money on an over the corner soap. Instead, you can buy soap from any local drug store. For me Oil of Olay works wonders. Plus, you also want to make sure that you use a good moisturizer. You will want to make this a daily routine at least once a day.

Cleaning your face at least once a day and moisturizing will help clear your skin and help heal any imperfections and blemishes you may have. Try cleaning your face before you brush your teeth this will definitely help. Also, I would look into adding any additional cleaners to this regiment, but don't ever do it. You want to use the right combination of soap, cleaner, and moisturize, you don't want to rip your skin of its natural glow. For the right combination consult a dermatologist. Having clear skin is indeed a battle, but it is a war that you can win.

The second tip is never pick or try to pop the blemish this will only make things worse. By trying to pop a blemish you can actually do serious damage that can damage the skin and ultimately lead to scarring. Treating the blemish and allowing your pores to breathe is the goal you will want to either try some ice or the cleaning method I mentioned earlier. If these imperfections or blemishes are more intense, then you should consult your doctor or dermatologist.

Now that you have started to solve the problem and begun the war against blemishes you can start to apply makeup in a healthy manner. The next step is to use the right concealer. You don't want to necessarily buy the most expensive one on the market, but you also don't want to buy the cheapest one either. This step may actually take a bit of trial and error to find the right one that fits your skin best. Remember you don't want to get frustrated.

Another tip you should definitely try is using a brush instead of your fingers or hands to blend in your concealer or foundation. By using a brush you will avoid getting any bacteria that may be on your hands and fingers on your face. By blending you will also cover the blemish in a smoother fashion. Another small tip is less more. Don't feel like you need to pour the makeup on your face to cover something up. If you use too much makeup you can actually make things worse by clogging up the pores and making it more difficult to clean.

Another tip is the foundation itself, if you have dry skin; I suggest using a cream based foundation. This is also another tip that can also be a trial and error situation. You may find that you need to try several different brands before finding the right one. I use a cream foundation and find that it's the best for me. Don't feel that because your mother used a brand for years that you have to follow suit. Find the right foundation that is right for you. By using a cream as a pose to a powder foundation you are actually helping your pores breathe easier.

Now it may seem like I'm trying to shy you away from powder completely this is not the case. You can indeed use powder, but try to avoid using powder as your base foundation. You can use powder to give you a healthy glow and shine, the look I'm sure you're going for.

Another tip is to try using liquid eyeliner, in case if you have yet to notice liquid is indeed the theme of this chapter. Using liquid eyeliner will help if you have dry skin. Use these instead of eye pencils to avoid drying out the skin even more.

We have learned that blemishes are a part of our lives, but you can follow these steps to create a beautiful healthy glow to your skin. Remember cleaning and cleansing is extremely important. Using the right product can help reduce and sometimes eliminate imperfections and blemishes. We have also mentioned that you cannot get too stressed or frustrated by these imperfections. This will make things worse. Finally, you've learned that using the right brand of foundation and type of foundation is important as well as the right way to apply these products. Remember there are a lot of methods around regarding how to treat the skin, but using these methods and techniques can help you not only get the skin you want, but apply the right product so you can put your best foot forward. Clear skin and applying makeup can be a battle, but now you have the tools to win the war. I hope these tips help.

CHAPTER 5- HOW TO APPLY FOUNDATION AND POWDER CORRECTLY

For years now, you have simply been in love with makeup. You are intrigued by the various application methods that people use, and you love to stay on top of new styles, trends and products. Despite your affection for makeup, you are not quite sure how to apply foundation and powder correctly. Since these are essentials, learning the basics is quite important.

Choosing the Right Products

Before you can apply the products correctly, you need to be sure that you have the right ones on-hand. Going to a store where you can actually try the foundation and powder on is most advisable. Otherwise, you could end up with colors that are not right for you. Colors that are too dark can actually make your face look dirty or over-tanned. Selecting shades that are too light might mean that you do not receive any coverage at all.

Selecting the Right Application Tools

Now that you have the foundation and loose powder in your hands, you must also obtain the right tools with which to apply them. Generally, opting for less expensive brushes is fine, and you can still obtain a flawless look with them. A big powder brush works best for your powder application as it helps to ensure an even distribution. This can also be used as a blending tool. As far as the foundation, you have a couple of different options. Wedge-shaped sponges tend to work well, and we will discuss the use of fingers for application in the next section.

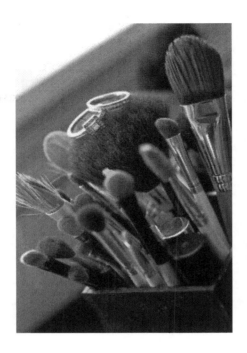

Using Your Fingers to Apply Foundation

Some people say that this is the best way to apply foundation. One of the perks is that you won't waste as much makeup. When you use a sponge, a decent amount of the foundation is absorbed as per the purpose of a sponge. You may end up having to replace your foundation more often than you would like. With your fingers, you would put a few dots on your face-generally on your forehead, cheeks and chin-and then work to blend them together. Try out different methods to see what works for you.

The Amount to Use

Many women do not know how much foundation and powder they should be using. Some of them don't use enough, and they wind up with practically no coverage at all. However, most of the problems come from the other end of the spectrum: women who go overboard with the product. When you are applying your makeup, you should start out with a small amount. You can start on your problem areas first and then blend to the other parts of your face. The amount of foundation you put on the sponge could be the size of a nickel, and you'll likely get a decent amount of coverage out of it. Then, you can add more as necessary.

Let Your Foundation Dry!

Here is where a lot of people make a big mistake. When you first put your foundation on, your skin is going to be a little bit wet. Just like paint, it needs time to dry before you put anything on top of that. Start to work on your hair or go pack up your bag while your foundation is drying on your face. Usually, just five minutes or so will do the trick. If you put powder on top of wet foundation, you are going to end up with a streaky and gooey mess.

Loose Powder as a Setter

Some women tend to use loose powder as another layer of foundation, and this is not quite what it was intended for. Yes, it does help to give you more coverage and to provide a flawless look to your face. However, it also helps to set the makeup and to make you appear polished. After the foundation application, your flaws should be covered for the most part. A few nice swipes of loose powder over your face will give your skin that even loose it deserves.

Applying Your Other Products

Remember, you need these products to work with your other makeup items as well. Put a little bit of foundation on your eyelids can work as a nice base for powder eye shadows. As with the loose powder, foundation must dry before you apply eye shadow. Just be careful to not get any of it in your eyes! Are you going to be wearing bronzer and blush as well? Once all of the products are on, use your big brush to enjoy that everything is completely blended together.

A Few Notes on Tinted Moisturizer

Every time you go into the foundation aisle at your local store, you seem some tinted moisturizer. You're curious to know more about these types of products. Well, they are great alternatives to foundation if you do not need a lot of coverage for your skin. Basically, they provide your skin with the moisture that it needs, but they also do give you a little bit of coverage. Some of them might have pink undertones, and others may help to give you a bit of a tan. They vary in their designs and forms, but they work to serve a similar function: coverage without that "heavy" feeling.

Ladies have plenty of options to explore when it comes to the world of foundations and powders. After selecting the right products, you'll now know how to put them on your face in the correct manner.

CHAPTER 6- EYE MAKEUP- SELECTION AND APPLICATION

So many different types of makeup exist, and you probably want a chance to experiment with them all. Well, eye makeup is one of those types, and an array of products is available on the market. With all of these choices, you might become overwhelmed. How can you tell the right way to pick out and apply makeup?

Consider Your Skin

In the preliminary stages of your eye makeup-selection research, you absolutely need to take your skin into account. If you are a person who has a lot of allergies, bringing your list of allergens to the store with you is imperative. Basically, people tend to get bad allergic reactions in your eyes. Using eye products to which you are allergic can be so harmful. On the other end of the spectrum, people who have oily skin will likely need a base for the eye makeup to cling to.

Make a List of Products

Once you have put together the various products and ingredients to which you might be allergic, you also need to make a list of exactly what you need. When it comes to eye makeup, eyeliner, mascara and eye shadow are generally considered to be the three basics. Eye shadow gives your lids a pop of color, and other two products really help them to stand out on your face. You may also opt for a primer as well. Primer can help your eye shadow to stay put all throughout the day and night.

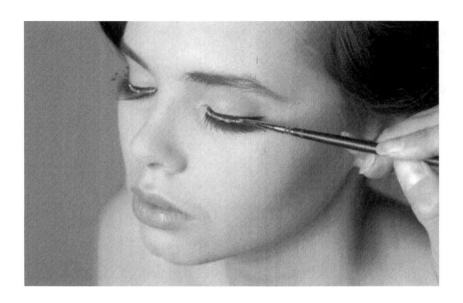

Creams, Powders and Liquid Liners

When you really start to research products, you're going to see that it is much more complicated that just a few simple categories. With eye shadows, you can select from creams or powders. Cream-based shades tend to pack a lot of power, and they can provide you with that dewey look that many ladies crave. However, they can also slide off easily. Powders generally tend to have more staying power, but you could combine the two for a really intriguing look. Eyeliners are often available in either pencil or liquid form. Liquid liners are usually more dramatic, but if you aren't careful, they could start dripping down your face early in the day.

The Colors to Use

Let's start with a discussion of eyeliner and mascara. Black eyeliner and mascara are generally considered to be the most dramatic. Of course, all different types and styles exist. Just because you wear black does not mean you need to look as though you are about to appear in a Broadway production. Still, if you want a more muted style, you could opt for brown liner and mascara. For those who are really new to makeup, clear mascara can lengthen and add volume to your lashes without any color at all.

Colors Continued: Picking Your Eye Shadow

Once you have the right shades for these two basics, you can start to look into eye shadow colors. Some people say the shadow should match your eye color, and others disagree. If you have blue eyes and swear blue shadow all over your lids, crease and brow bone, it probably won't work too well. However, blending the blue with a cream or white can create a delicate look that's really pretty. Look for kits that contain great colors for certain eye types to ensure you have an arsenal of supplies.

Covering the Lid

When you put on eye shadow, your lid of your eye is the biggest part. Now, plenty of different ways exist to do makeup. However, in order to break the rules of makeup application and know your own path, knowing a fairly basic pattern is important. Once you master this, you can start to get creative. Start with three colors that are in the same family. Take the medium one and use a flat brush to cover your entire lid with it. Pay special attention to the crease as this is where shadow can start to fall off.

The Other Two Colors

What should you do with the other two colors in the kit? Use the darkest one to fill in the crease even more. You should be blending this with the middle shade to ensure that it looks smooth and professional. As for the lightest color, you can blend that up to your brow bone. Consider where you are going as you apply these colors. For a day at the office, the lid color might be just enough. When you are going out with the girls, get a little fancier and try all three of them.

Other Tips and Hints

Using an eyelash curler can definitely bring you some extra appeal, so don't be afraid to employ its power. Before you put any makeup on your eyelids, you need to make sure they are dry. Otherwise, the makeup is going to fall off. You should remember that if you put eyeliner on after your eye shadow, it will look better. If you do not, the shadow will just cover up the liner. Keep a cotton swab on hand, especially when you are applying the mascara. If anything gets messy or all over the place, you can just wipe that bit off instead of having to start all over.

Selecting and applying eye makeup can seem a little bit overwhelming to someone who has never done it before. Fortunately, once you start to get the hang of it, you'll begin to feel like a professional makeup artist.

CHAPTER 7- MAKEUP APPLICATION- HOW TO APPLY LIPSTICK

Beautiful lips are a goal of many, and you certainly have your eyes set on a prettier pucker. For years now, you have been playing around with glosses and the like, but you are ready to move on to lipstick. What do you need to know about the application of this product?

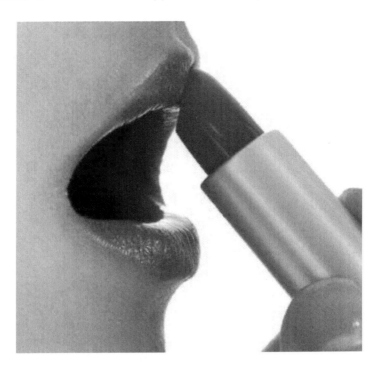

Choosing the Right Lipstick for You

No matter what you do, you aren't going to have gorgeous, glowing lips if you choose a shade that does not work for you. You do not necessarily have to pick the most expensive product on the market, but you should look into quality items. You don't want ones that are going to break or be rendered useless after they have been utilized for only a short period of time. Select shades that work with your skin but that also complement the colors of makeup you tend to wear out.

Preparing Your Lips for Application

Even if you picked out the most gorgeous color in the world from the fanciest line of makeup ever, you could still look un-groomed if you do not prepare your lips for the process. After you brush your teeth, you should use a toothbrush with warm water on it only to gently scrub your lips. This helps to get rid of dead skin on them and to make them much smoother. As soon as you are done, use a nice lip balm. Always keep your lips moisturized, or they might crack when you put on lipstick.

Be Careful of Super Drying Lipsticks

As you probably have already surmised on your own, lipsticks tend to be drier than lip glosses. Not all lipsticks have that balm-like quality to them, and, as a result, even the softest of lips might be subject to cracking and peeling. You need to look for the ingredients in the lipstick, but you also must be wary of certain types. For example, have you seen any of those lipsticks on the market that promise to last all day long? These tend to sting a little bit and to really dry out your kisser.

Using Lip Liner to Enhance Your Lips

Before you can put on the lipstick, you need to use a lip liner to really provide that perfect appeal. First, you should choose a lip liner that goes with the lipstick you have selected. Trying a few different types at the store would be the smartest thing. Of course, the liner should be in the same color family, and it would be best if the two were as close as possible. Otherwise, you lips might look very fake and overdone. Work to keep the lip liner as close to the actual line of your lips as possible.

That First Coat

Generally, you want to take the lipstick to the middle of your bottom lip and the middle of your top lip first. If you wish, you could use the liner on your lip before that, but it's not really necessary. Remember, lipstick is easy to reapply, so you do not absolutely need it to last all day. As long as you have the lipstick and a mirror with you, you are good to go. Once you have the first coat neatly on, without going past the liner of course, you can rub your lips together a little bit.

Can I Add More?

Now that you have put the first coat of your lipstick on, you can work to add a little bit more to your smile. Waiting for it to dry a bit is a smart idea. Otherwise, you may just end up smudging the lipstick around and not really achieving the look that you have desired. Not only can the lipstick smudge and become messy, but it might also start to just look way too intense. You want to use makeup to enhance your look, not to take it over.

Add the Finishing Touches

Lipstick should not take a very long time to apply. At this point, you are probably ready to go. If the color is too overwhelming right now, you can use a tissue to blot it. This ensures that the color stays on but not in such an intense amount. Sometimes, lipstick can make your lips look a little bit too dry. If that is the case, you could always add a bit of clear gloss on top. When you have a gloss that matches the color of your lipstick, this might work as well. Just don't add on a ton, or you'll end up with that "overdone" look.

Reapplying Your Lipstick

Unless you use one of those super-staying lipsticks, you are going to have to reapply at some point during the day. Even when you use those tips, a lot of talking, eating or drinking can still start to wear away at them. Just be sure to have all of your products on you. If you just bring the lipstick and not the liner, you might not look quite the same later on in the evening. When you want tips and tricks on how to make the look last longer, consider consulting with a professional makeup artist.

Makeup is certainly enjoyable to play with, but it is not all fun and games. Using some specific tips to help you achieve lovely lips is really going to make you love looking in the mirror when you are out.

ABOUT THE AUTHOR

Lisa Patrick loves everything natural and is a bit of a health nut but she also loves makeup and loves to give persons advice on how to apply it properly. She learned how to do the basics from her mother and improved upon her technique by watching videos and going to a few courses on makeup application. With the encouragement of her friends, she made the decision to do a set of books that would help other women to learn how to apply makeup the right way.

Lisa highlights the different looks that women can have when they go to work or go to a wedding. She even has a bit of advice for those females that have problem with their skin. When the reader has completed the book they will even have some tips on how to have a younger or older look depending on the age they are.

Made in the USA
Lexington, KY
25 June 2016